TABLE OF CONTENTS

CHAPTER 01

WHY I STOPPED YOGA

I'm excited to share with you a topic that has become incredibly important to me: joint hypermobility. I've spent years in the fitness world, first as a Pilates instructor, then dabbled in Yoga and Hot Yoga for years, and then returned to being a dedicated Pilates practitioner and a Masseuse.

I've experienced and witnessed firsthand the unique challenges that hypermobility presents. This book is my way of addressing those challenges and offering solutions to help others navigate their fitness journeys safely.

For those who might not be familiar with the term, hypermobility is a condition where the joints can move beyond the typical range of motion. You might be more familiar with the term double-jointed.

While this might sound like an advantage, it can pose significant risks, particularly in certain types of exercise. This condition ranges in degrees, so the misconception is that many do not realise they are as it does not present as extreme as expected. You might not have discomfort, but in some cases, after years of extreme range, you present with tightness in that area, or in other words, hypomobility.

My journey to practising yoga was initially a business decision. I was a passionate Pilates instructor when I was repeatedly asked to cover Yoga classes. Initially, I was hesitant because Yoga and Pilates, though both valuable, are fundamentally different.

Yoga is rooted in ancient Hindu spiritual practices. Moreover, not all styles suit everyone, especially those with hypermobility.

I didn't understand this at the time. However, being a Christian is a significant reason not to have started. Sadly, my peers had not explained why, so I just went ahead without researching. I just assumed it was safe to learn from a fitness point of view.

Having progressed to become qualified also to teach Hot Yoga, I soon realised that Yoga poses, particularly in heated environments, be it Hot Yoga or Bikram, could lead to overstretching without realising, resulting in joint instability or even injury.

Many are unaware of their 'range of movement' and, as a consequence, don't know their limits, especially when stretching. If this is the case in normal temperatures, imagine what that means in the comfort of a heated room!

As an instructor for many years, I've encountered countless clients whose issues could be traced back to their Yoga practice. Some had difficulty getting to the floor, bending their knees, and moving their necks fully. These issues are often exacerbated by exercise routines not properly executed or overstretching. The most concerning cases I noted were of students with hypermobility, who end up with debilitating injuries following sessions and struggle to do daily activities as a result.

This book is born out of a desire to offer a safer, more effective alternative for those with hypermobility, and all others who are genuinely interested in fitness. Pilates focuses on strength, stability, and correct alignment, which sets a controlled environment where individuals can build muscle and protect joints. In contrast, there are definite risks associated with forms of Yoga.

While Yoga prioritises flexibility at the expense of stability, Pilates emphasises core engagement and alignment, making it an excellent choice for those with hypermobility.

Throughout my career, I've seen incredible transformations in clients who exchanged Yoga for Pilates. They became stronger, more stable, and deeply aware of their body, requiring fewer treatments for pain and injury. This book is my way of sharing these insights and helping fitness enthusiasts avoid the pitfalls I've come across and have experienced personally.

For individuals with hypermobility, who are seeking an approach to stay active without risking health to their joints, I urge them to explore Pilates. Exercise should not be about pushing the body to its limits but finding a balance that respects the body's unique capabilities and capacities. You will see a difference in your joints and overall well-being..

In writing this book, my goal is to educate and empower those with hypermobility to make informed choices about their fitness routines. By choosing Pilates, you could protect yourself from unnecessary injuries and build a stronger, healthier body. So, roll out your mat, engage your core, and let's embark on this journey to strength and stability together.

CHAPTER 02

WHAT IS JOINT HYPERMOBILITY?

As an instructor for 14 years, I've had the privilege of seeing how exercise can profoundly impact lives. I have also witnessed challenges that arise, especially for individuals with Hypermobility issues. While this condition may seem like a gift, it can present unique obstacles on the fitness journey. And believe me, I have learnt from my personal experience. When it comes to managing hypermobility, not all exercises are created equal.

As mentioned previously, hypermobility refers to a condition where an individual's joints can move beyond the normal range of motion. This may sound impressive; however, it could actually be a double-edged sword, particularly in activities like Yoga.

I discovered this firsthand when I was asked on several occasions to cover Yoga classes at a busy city gym where I primarily taught Pilates. Initially, I hesitated.

Despite my background in Pilates, Yoga was a completely different discipline. In my head then, it was not as exciting as Pilates and was actually too static and slow, verging on the borderline of 'boring'. I am aware that some Yogis might think the same of Pilates, too!

Pilates, on the other hand, instantly resonated with me as an exercise routine. I felt energised, and my back felt fantastic immediately! However, it also highlighted my weakness in upper body extremities and poor circulation, as I got leg cramps during classes initially.

Eventually, I took on more work, which meant deeper stretches and dynamic movements. I felt weaker in some joints and tighter around my hips, which didn't make sense, so I did more to try and alleviate those symptoms. When teaching, I remained cautious, especially when working with those who were hypermobile.

During my instructor training course, I remember the trainer not wanting me to focus on positioning. She said, "We are all freaks," meaning we cannot aim to perfect the poses. With Pilates, an instructor is expected to give cues to correct position and transitions.

In contrast, I was being told to disregard discipline. This shocked me, as the trainer was a master trainer and someone I regarded highly. This, for me, concludes the main differences between the two disciplines. I was always going to teach grounded in my Pilates foundation anyway. This was another reason to prompt me to open my own studio.

For individuals with hypermobile joints, it's incredibly easy to overstretch without even realising it. This could lead to a range of complications, from bursitis, minor sprains, and strains to more serious problems like joint instability, dislocations, and more.

Pilates is an excellent option for individuals with hypermobility because it focuses on building strength and stability in a controlled environment. Unlike Yoga, which can sometimes prioritise flexibility above all else, Pilates emphasises proper alignment and core engagement.

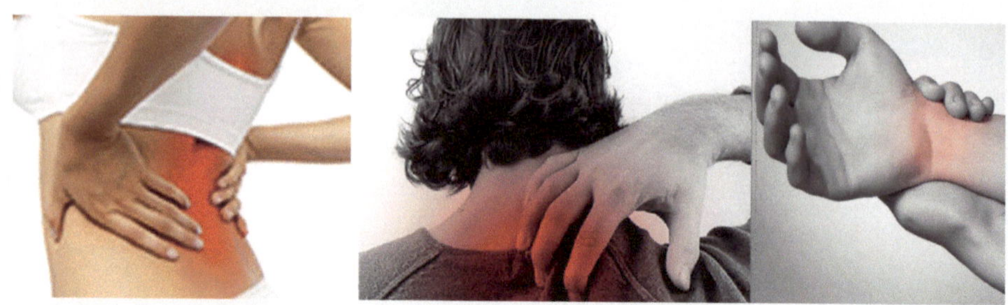

This approach helps prevent overstretching and reduces the risk of injury. I've seen incredible transformations in clients who have made the switch from Yoga to Pilates. They have become stronger, more stable and more in tune with their bodies. Many have reported needing fewer treatments and have developed a heightened sense of body awareness. It's truly remarkable how the right exercise regime can enhance overall well-being.

If you have hypermobility and are seeking a safer way to stay fit and healthy, I strongly recommend giving Pilates a try. It is not about pushing yourself to the limit in every session; it is about finding a balance that works for your body and honours its unique needs. Trust me, your joints will thank you in the long run.

Yoga injuries are a real concern for individuals with Hypermobility, and by switching to Pilates, you can protect yourself from unnecessary sprains, strains, and joint issues. So, roll out that Pilates mat, engage your core, and let's work together to strengthen those muscles and joints. Your body will thank you for prioritising strength, stability, and safety.

CHAPTER 03

PILATES VS YOGA - THE BASICS

When it comes to choosing between Pilates and Yoga, it's essential to understand their distinct origins, philosophies, and physical benefits. Both practices are highly regarded for their mind-body connection, focus on breath, and ability to improve overall well-being, but they cater to different needs and goals.

Origins and Philosophy Pilates:

Developed by: Joseph Pilates in the early 20th century.

Purpose: Originally designed as a rehabilitation method for injured soldiers during World War I, Pilates focuses on controlled movements to strengthen the "Powerhouse," which includes the core, back, hips, and glutes.

Approach: Pilates is highly structured and emphasises precision, control, and stability. The exercises are often done on a mat or specialised equipment like the Reformer or Cadillac, designed to enhance muscle tone and stability.

Physical Benefits Pilates:

Core Strength: Pilates is renowned for its focus on building a strong core, which supports the spine and improves overall stability.

Posture and Alignment: By emphasising precise movements, Pilates helps improve posture and realign the body, often leading to a feeling of increased, reduced back pain, and rehabilitation.

Yoga: Developed over 5,000 years ago in India.

Purpose: Yoga is a spiritual Hindu practice dating back thousands of years. Yoga is a practice that encompasses not only physical postures (asanas) but also meditation, breath work (pranayama). It's designed to prepare the body and mind for prolonged meditation as the spiritual aspect of Yoga is central.

Approach: Yoga offers a broad spectrum of practices, from physically demanding (like Ashtanga) to meditative (like Yin or Hatha). The spiritual aspect of yoga is central, with a focus on achieving balance and harmony between mind, body, and spirit.

Contrast:
 Due to its controlled, low-impact nature, Pilates is often used in physical therapy to help with injury recovery and prevention.

Flexibility: Yoga focuses on flexibility. Heated classes, like Bikram, encourage deeper stretches and holding poses for extended periods.

 Researchgate shows 62% of survey participants had suffered one or more musculoskeletal injuries that lasted in excess of one month. The three most common injury locations were hamstring, knee, and low back in Vinyasa or Ashtanga yoga

Mind-Body Connection: Yoga emphasises on breath and meditation.

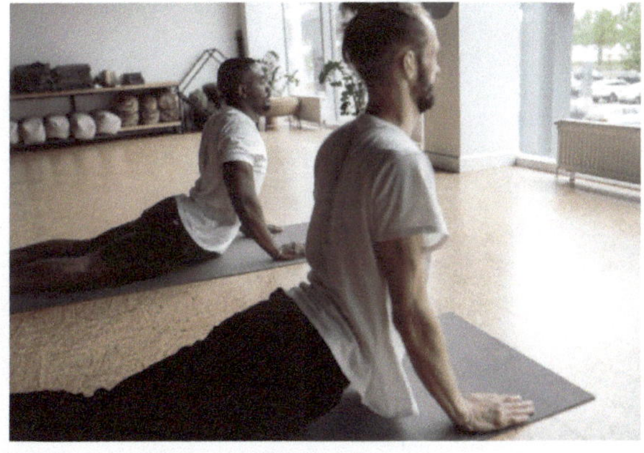

Choosing Between Pilates & Yoga:

Both Pilates and yoga can be beginner-friendly, but the choice depends on your goals. If you're looking to build core strength and improve posture with added flexibility and relaxation, Pilates might be the better option. If you seek flexibility, relaxation, and a Hindu spirituality component, Yoga may be more suitable.

Complementing Other Workouts:

Pilates can complement strength training by enhancing core stability and flexibility, as well as energising and encouraging happy endorphins, while Yoga can focus on flexibility and mental focus.

Final thoughts: Ultimately, Pilates has a wider range of benefits and is a safer practice. Your choice should be guided by your personal goals, preferences, and any existing physical conditions.

CHAPTER 04

THE IMPORTANCE
OF BREATHING

This chapter will explore the fundamental importance of efficient respiration and shed light on how conscious breathing practices can positively impact our physical health and vitality.

In today's fast-paced world, we often take the simple act of breathing for granted. We breathe in oxygen and exhale carbon dioxide without much thought, but the process of respiration is far more intricate than it appears on the surface.

The primary purpose of breathing is to supply oxygen to our cells, aid in energy production, and facilitate various essential cellular reactions that are crucial for our bodies to function effectively.

However, people often fail to realise that the efficiency of the breathing process hinges on the balance of carbon dioxide in our bodies.

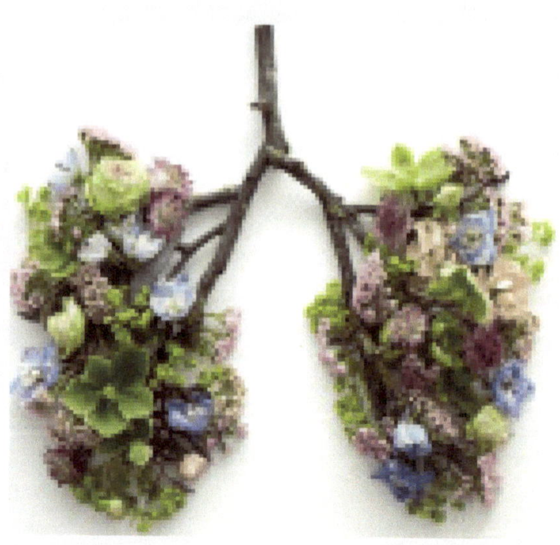

While oxygen is vital, an adequate level of carbon dioxide is equally important for optimal respiration. Without this delicate equilibrium, our bodies may face various challenges, including decreased energy production and potential long-term health issues.

In the quest to maintain a healthy and active lifestyle, it is crucial to understand the significance of proper breathing techniques. By delving deeper into the mechanics of respiration and its role in supporting cellular energy production, individuals can take proactive steps to prevent potential injuries and safeguard their overall well-being.

Over time, I noticed a common pattern among individuals with hypermobility, including myself, was the tendency to brace. This involves holding one's breath and/or tensing the body in an attempt to create stability.

Normal breathing requires the use of our diaphragm and intercostal muscles also known as the primary respiratory muscles. Sadly, the shallow breathers have worse side effects. If the primary breathing muscles do not engage, it forces the secondary muscles to work.

These include the upper Trapezius, Scalene, sternocleidomastoid, levator scapulae, and pectoralis minor. The required effort to be activated, which in turn, can cause adverse underlining issues to your alignment in the long term.

Certain styles of Yoga, such as hot Yoga or Bikram, can exacerbate risks to joints. Hot yoga was the training I took as it was regulated properly and considered a safe temperature, unlike the extremes Bikram took. Some even fainted in some sessions, as shown in the Netflix documentary if you were not aware!

Individuals are encouraged to breathe deeply and meditate as a fundamental concept of Yoga. The intense heat in these sessions could make individuals feel more flexible than they actually are, tempting them to push their bodies beyond safe limits.

Within the context of hypermobility, deep breathing could sometimes lead to hypoxia, a condition where too little oxygen reaches the brain and muscles due to excessive inhalation and reduced carbon dioxide levels. This could create a sensation that is often mistaken for the calm, meditative state yoga seeks to achieve, but in reality, it may be causing localised pain and discomfort.

CHAPTER 05

HYPERMOBILES BEWARE:
RISKS OF YOGA

By highlighting the importance of approaching physical activity with caution and awareness, this chapter aims to empower hypermobile individuals to make informed choices that prioritise their long-term well-being. Promoting Pilates as a mindful, controlled, and safer alternative for hypermobile individuals underscores the significance of choosing practices that support joint health and overall stability.

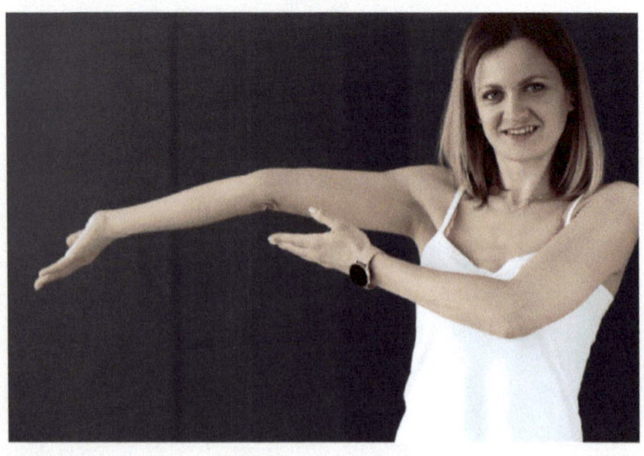

Individuals who possess hypermobility face unique challenges when it comes to physical activity, particularly in practices like yoga. While flexibility is often celebrated in yoga, hypermobile individuals must be cautious of the risks associated with hyperextension and locking joints in certain poses.

 The excessive range of movement that comes with hypermobility can compromise joint stability, increasing the likelihood of injuries and chronic pain.

In contrast to the emphasis on flexibility in Yoga, Pilates prioritises stability and strength-building to support the body's natural alignment and functionality. Hypermobile individuals may find that controlled movements and a focus on core engagement in Pilates provide a safer and more sustainable approach to exercise.

Through personal experiences and anecdotes, I have come to understand that hypermobility could be misunderstood in Yoga sessions, leading to unintended injuries and life-changing setbacks. By advocating for informed modifications and safe movement practices, hypermobile individuals could navigate their physical practice with greater awareness and care. Some instructors wrongly cue 'Lock your knees for example'! An absolute NO NO!

Selecting movement modalities that prioritise joint protection and strength building is essential for hypermobile individuals to prevent exacerbating existing issues.

SACROILIAC JOINT DYSFUNCTION AND LOW BACK PAIN

This chapter aims to empower readers to make informed decisions about their movement practices.

SI joint dysfunction and low back pain are common issues that many individuals encounter, especially those who engage in physical practices like yoga. The repetitive movements involved in yoga, coupled with Hypermobility, could put a strain on the sacroiliac joint, leading to discomfort and potential dysfunction issues.

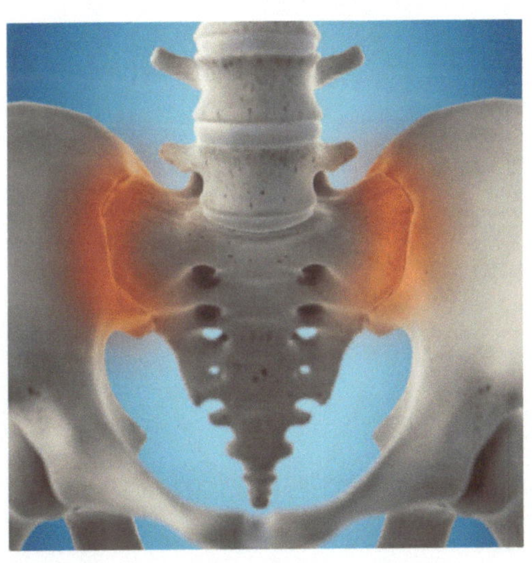

To address these concerns effectively, it is crucial to have a comprehensive understanding of the biomechanics of the SI joint and how it contributes to back pain.

Incorrect alignment and movements in yoga practices can exacerbate SI joint issues, highlighting the need for a mindful approach to movement to protect joint health.

Research studies have shed light on the prevalence of SI joint dysfunction among Yoga practitioners, emphasising the importance of awareness and proper technique in preventing injury.

Personal experiences and case studies further underscore the real-life implications of SI joint pain resulting from Yoga practice, prompting individuals to re-evaluate their movement choices.

To address these concerns effectively, it is crucial to have a comprehensive understanding of the biomechanics of the SI joint and how it contributes to backpain. Incorrect alignment and movements in Yoga practices can exacerbate SI joint issues, highlighting the need for a mindful approach to movement to protect joint health.

In contrast, Pilates offers a beneficial alternative for stabilising the SI joint and mitigating back pain through targeted exercises and core strengthening techniques.

An evidence-based approach to addressing sacroiliac joint issues through Pilates not only provides relief but also promotes long-term joint health and well-being.

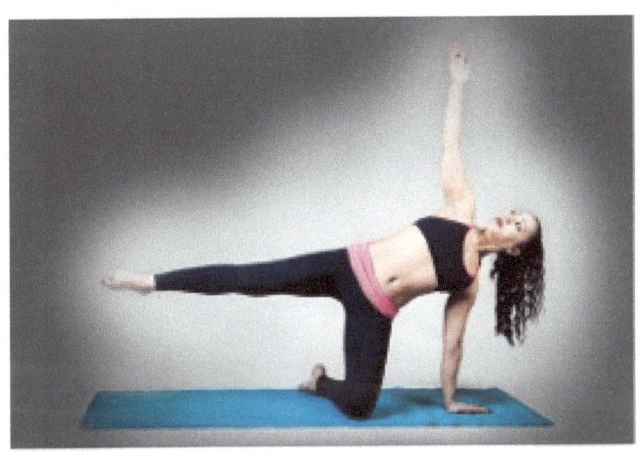

Comparing the effectiveness of Yoga and Pilates in strengthening the core to support the SI joint reveals the advantages of Pilates in fostering stability and resilience. By offering resources and information for individuals seeking relief from SI joint dysfunction and low back pain through Pilates

Ultimately, encouraging a mindful and safe approach to movement is key to promoting SI joint health and overall well-being, highlighting the importance of selecting practices that prioritise joint stability and functional strength.

CHAPTER 07

PILATES AS A SAFER ALTERNATIVE

One of the key benefits of Pilates is its ability to develop strength and body awareness, enhancing overall physical functionality and movement efficiency. This is particularly relevant for hypermobile individuals, as Pilates emphasis on stability and controlled strength can provide a supportive framework for managing Hypermobility and preventing injury.

Success stories of individuals who have transitioned from Yoga to Pilates highlight the transformative impact of this shift. By leveraging statistics on the safety record of Pilates compared to Yoga, it becomes clear that Pilates offers a lower-risk option for individuals seeking a sustainable and injury-resistant form of exercise.

Pilates stands out as a safe and effective movement practice that prioritises alignment, core stability, and controlled movements. Unlike Yoga, which may carry a higher riskof injury dueto its emphasison extreme flexibility and challenging poses, Pilates focuses on injury prevention through mindful and purposeful movements.

Through examples of Pilates exercises that promote strength, stability, and overall wellness, individuals can gain insight into the practical applications of this movement modality. By illustrating how Pilates supportsjoint health and helps prevent long-term injuries, this chapter underscores the holistic benefits of Pilates as a valuable alternative to Yoga practice.

Ultimately, readers are encouraged to consider Pilates as a comprehensive and effective approach to movement that not only enhances physical fitness but also promotes long-term health and well-being.

By embracing the principles of Pilates, individuals can cultivate a strong, stable foundation for sustainable movement practices and optimal body function.

CHAPTER 08

HOW PILATES SUPPORTS HYPERMOBILE INDIVIDUALS

In the realm of movement practices, Pilates emerges as a valuable tool for hypermobile individuals seeking stability and joint support. Through its emphasis on controlled movements, Pilates offers a structured approach to prevent hyperextension and protect vulnerable joints from excessive strain.

Unlike Yoga, where the focus on extreme flexibility can pose risks for hypermobile individuals, Pilates strikes a balance between developing strength and maintaining flexibility.

One of the key distinguishing factors of Pilates is its focus on core engagement, which plays a pivotal role in supporting the entire body and minimising the chances of injury. By honing in on alignment and correct form, Pilates practitioners cultivate a strong foundation that promotes optimal movement mechanics and joint integrity.

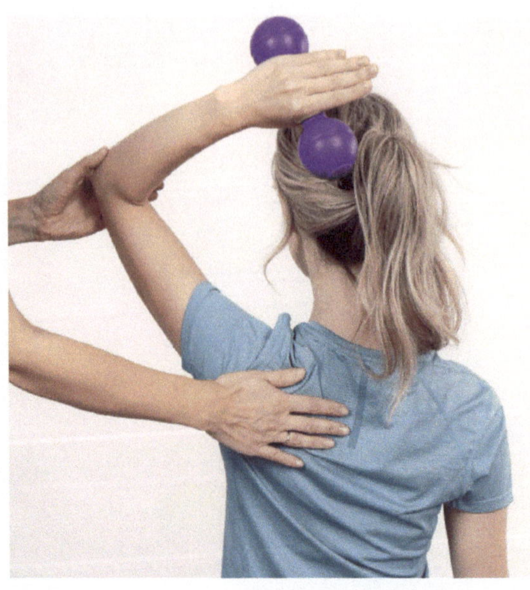

CHAPTER 09

THE SCIENCE BEHIND MOVEMENT: PILATES VS. YOGA

Personal testimonies from hypermobile individuals thriving in Pilates sessions confirm the transformative impact of this discipline on joint health and overall well-being. Pilates not only aids in physical strength but also enhances body awareness and perception, allowing individuals to move with mindfulness and precision.

Scientific research further solidifies the efficacy of Pilates for hypermobility, highlighting its ability to improve joint stability and functional movement capacity. By encouraging Hypermobile individuals to explore Pilates as a safe and tailored movement practice, this book aims to empower them to prioritise joint health and injury prevention in their fitness journey. Through Pilates, individuals can harness their unique abilities and navigate physical activity with confidence, ensuring long-term well-being and resilience.

When comparing Pilates and Yoga, it is essential to understand the contrasting anatomical principles and movements emphasised in each practice.

While Yoga often focuses on flexibility and flowing movements, Pilatesprioritises core engagement and controlled, precise movements. This distinction plays a significant role in how each practice approaches strength, flexibility, and overall body awareness.

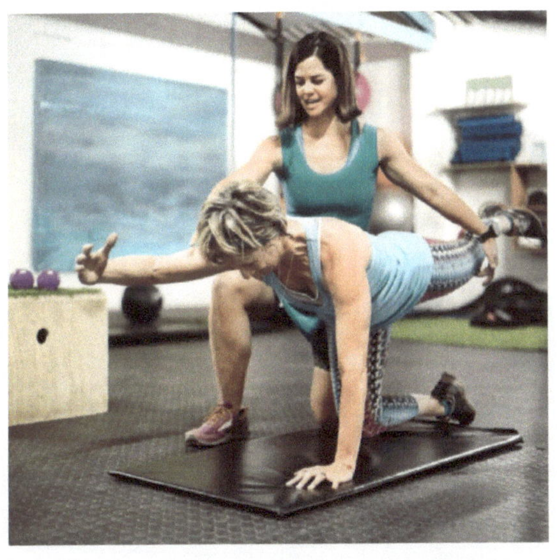

Core engagement and stabilisation techniques differ between Pilates and Yoga, with Pilates placing a strong emphasis on activating the core muscles to support the spine and stabilise the body during movements.

In contrast, Yoga may incorporate more dynamic movements and stretching exercises without the same level of focus on core stability.

Mindful movement and body awareness are integral components of both Pilates and Yoga, promoting a deeper connection between the mind and body during exercise. However, the potentialrisk of hyperextension and joint strain in certain Yoga postures is higher comparedto the controlled and alignment-focused approach of Pilates.

Statistical data on injury rates and safety records of Pilates versus Yoga highlight the lower incidence of injuries associated with Pilates, making it a safer option for individuals looking to prioritise long-term joint health and injury prevention.

By providing examples of exercises in Pilates that specifically target strength-building and stability, individuals should note the practical applications of this practice in enhancing physical fitness and well-being.

Additionally, studies supporting the role of Pilates in enhancing posture and alignment underscore its holistic approach to physical health.

Scientific research confirms the efficacy of Pilates for Hypermobility, highlighting its ability to improve joint stability and functional movement capacity. By encouraging Hypermobile individuals to explore Pilates as a safe and tailored movement practice, this book aims to empower individuals to prioritise joint health and injury prevention throughout their fitness journey. Through Pilates, individuals could harness unique abilities and navigate physical activity with confidence, ensuring long-term well-being and resilience.

By understanding the differences between Pilates and Yoga and recognising the therapeutic potential of Pilates for joint health and injury prevention, individuals could make empowered choices that support their long-term health and vitality.

Readers are encouraged to consider scientific evidence when selecting a movement practice for their holistic well-being, with an emphasis on the importance of making informed decisions that align with their individual needs and goals.

CHAPTER 10

INJURY PREVENTION: PILATES OVER YOGA

In today's fitness landscape, the risk of injuries in Yoga practices cannot be overlooked, as these injuries have the potential to cause long-term damage to the body. The dynamic and often demanding nature of Yoga poses can put stress on joints and muscles, leading to strains, sprains, and other traumatic injuries that may impact individuals for years to come.

In contrast, Pilates offers a safer alternative with its emphasis on proper alignment and controlled movements. By prioritising alignment and core stability, Pilates helps reduce the risk of injuries by fostering a more mindful and intentional approach to movement. This approach minimises the chances of overstraining muscles and joints, contributing to a lower rate of injuries compared to yoga.

Hypermobility can be misunderstood during Yoga sessions, leading to unintended injuries and setbacks. By advocating for informed modifications and safe movement practices, hypermobile individuals could navigate their physical practice with greater awareness and care.

Mindful movement and body awareness are integral components of both Pilates and Yoga, promoting a deeper connection between the mind and body during exercise. However, the potential risk of hyperextension and joint strain in certain Yoga postures is higher compared to the controlled and alignment-focused approach of Pilates.

Statistics on the prevalence of injuries in Yoga versus Pilates further highlight the importance of adopting a practice that prioritises injury prevention. Pilates' focuses on joint stability and muscle control which in turn plays a crucial role in safeguarding against injuries, as this encourages individuals to move with precision and awareness, reducing the likelihood of accidental harm.

Repetitive movements in Yoga can contribute to injury development over time, underscoring the need for a practice like Pilates that emphasises functional movement patterns and dynamic stability..

On the Pilates reformer, we have the safety of the pulleys assisting or the foot bar giving feedback and the shoulder rest protection from hunching the shoulder's to teach stability.

Case studies and research findings on the effectiveness of Pilates in injury prevention provide a scientific basis for the practice's impact on reducing the risk of injuries and promoting safe, sustainable movement habits.

By encouraging you to prioritise injury prevention and long-term well-being through Pilates practice, this chapter reinforces the importance of choosing a movement modality that supports overall health and longevity.

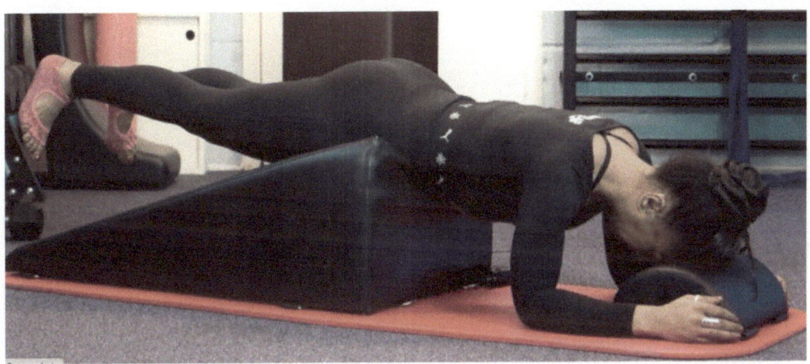

CHAPTER 11

PILATES FOR
HEALTHY FEET

Pilates exercises begin by lying on your back (supine)either on the floor or on a Reformer. This immediately takes the pressure off the spine and increases proprioception. When we cannot use our eyes to see the movement, mostly with our head down, we have to pay more attention to how it feels and use the 'Mind & Body' connection. We become 'core strong' before standing and working against gravity.

Moreover, using the footbar on the reformer enables us to strengthen our foot muscles, which need to be strengthened and worked on just like the rest of our body.

The foot functions as both an adjustable adapter and a rigid lever, facilitating movement from the moment of heel strike(deceleration) through mid-stance adjustments to the toe-off phase (acceleration). It plays a critical role in flexion, extension, adduction, abduction, and the tri-planar motions (rotation) of the subtalar joint.

These combined movements enable the full range of motion that we often take for granted, underscoring the complexity of the foot's structure.

The lower limb, extending from the knee to the foot, is not only crucial for extension, flexion, and support of foot movements, but also plays a vital role in the body's venous pump system. While the heart effectively pumps blood to the body's extremities, including the foot, the return of blood to the heart for reoxygenation is a more challenging task, particularly from the foot, the furthest and lowest extremity.

Unlike arteries, veins lack a dedicated pump to assist in this return. Instead, this function is primarily achieved through the action of the calf muscles, particularly the triceps surae group (gastrocnemius and soleus).
By contracting during movement and exercise, these muscles help overcome the challenges of distance and gravity, facilitating the return of blood to the heart.

Pilates offers significant benefits in maintaining and enhancing the function of these structures. It promotes increased blood circulation to and from the foot, ensuring a continuous supply of oxygen, energy, and nutrients to the lower limb while also aiding in the removal of toxins and carbon dioxide.

 Learning foot function through Pilates, particularly in a supine position, allows for more controlled and focused engagement of the foot and lower limb muscles without the added challenge of standing or balancing yoga poses, making it a more effective method for honing these specific movements and improving balance.

 Nearly every Pilates exercise involves pointing or flexing your feet. Footwork on the Reformer offers a unique and effective approach to improving foot and lower extremity biomechanics, as well as enhancing foot flexibility and strength. With consistent practice, Pilates can help alleviate and even eliminate foot pain.

 Pilates has even got a Foot and Toe correction devices to help focus Footwork more!

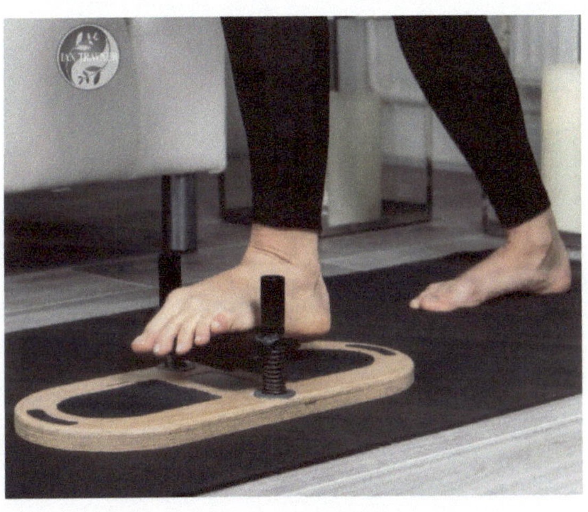

The advantages of Pilates for the lower limb and foot are multifaceted, particularly in terms of stretching. This is especially beneficial for the muscle layers of the sole, which act as a supportive strap, maintaining the integrity of the foot's arches and preventing collapse.

Overall, Pilates improves adaptability, articulation, and range of motion in the foot and lower limb. Additionally, enhanced blood circulation, which also contributes to improved respiratory function, highlights the extensive benefits that Pilates can provide.

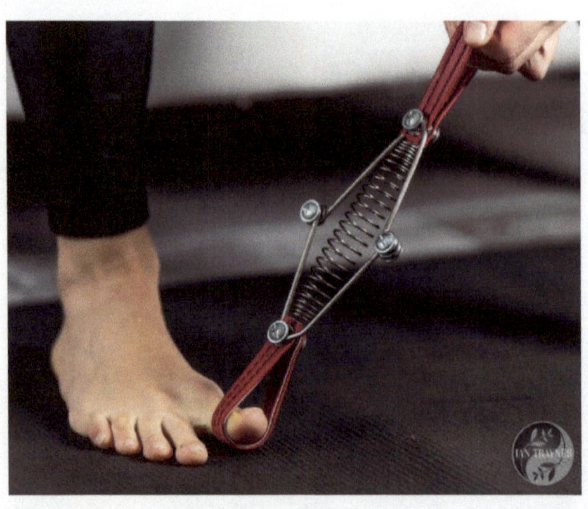

CHAPTER 12

TRANSITIONING FROM YOGA TO PILATES

Transitioning from a Yoga practice to Pilates is not just a change in workout routine; it is a shift towards overall wellness. Understanding the differences in movement principles between Yoga and Pilates is key to this transition. While Yoga often focuses on flexibility and flow, Pilates prioritises strength, stability, and controlled movements. This shift requires a guided approach to adapt from a flexibility-focused practice to a strength-building one.

Proper alignment and muscle engagement play a crucial role in Pilates, highlighting the importance of precision and control in movement.

As practitioners make the gradual shift from a mindset of relaxation in Yoga to one of active control in Pilates, they begin to understand the nuances of movement and the impact of focused, intentional exercises on their overall fitness.

Success stories of individuals who have made the switch from Yoga to Pilates serve as inspiring examples of the benefitsthat can be experienced through this transition. These individuals have found that Pilates not only enhances physical strength but also improves alignment, muscle engagement, and overall body awareness.

Readers are encouraged to consider Pilates as a comprehensive and effective approach to movement that not only enhances physical fitness but also promotes long-term health and well-being. By embracing the principles of Pilates, individuals can cultivate a strong, stable foundation for sustainable movement practices and optimal body function.

Personal stories from hypermobile individuals thriving in Pilates sessions confirm the transformative impact of this discipline on joint health and overall well-being.

Pilates aids physical strength and enhances body awareness and proprioception, allowing individuals to move with mindfulness and precision.

When comparing Pilates and Yoga, it is essential to understand the contrasting anatomical principles and movements emphasised within each practice. While Yoga often focuses on flexibility and flowing movements, Pilates prioritises core engagement and controlled, precise movements. This distinction plays a significant role in how each practice approaches strength, flexibility, and overall body awareness.

Core engagement and stabilisation techniques differ between Pilates and Yoga, with Pilates placing a strong emphasis on activating the core muscles to support the spine and stabilize the body during movements.

In contrast, Yoga may incorporate more dynamic movements and stretching exercises without the same level of focus on core stability.

Through examples which illustrate how Pilates promotes safer movement patterns, individuals could visualise the practical applications of this practicein preventing injuries and supporting overall physical health.

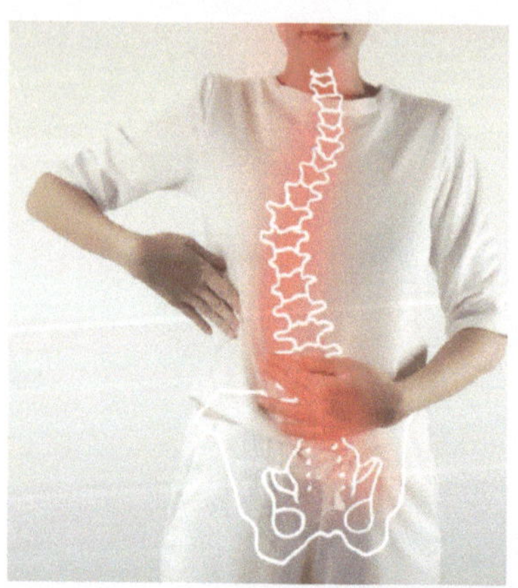

CHAPTER 13

PILATES EXERCISES FOR STRENGTH AND STABILITY

Pilates exercises are specifically designed to target core strength and stability, creating a strong foundation for overall physical fitness. By incorporating exercises that emphasise proper alignment and muscle engagement, Pilates practitioners could enhance body awareness and refine movement patterns to prevent injuries and improve functional capabilities.

In addition to core strength, Pilates exercises also focus on improving balance and perception, key components of physical fitness that contribute to stability and coordination. By incorporating Pilates equipment such as reformers or stability balls, individuals could introduce resistance and stability challenges to further enhance their workout routine.

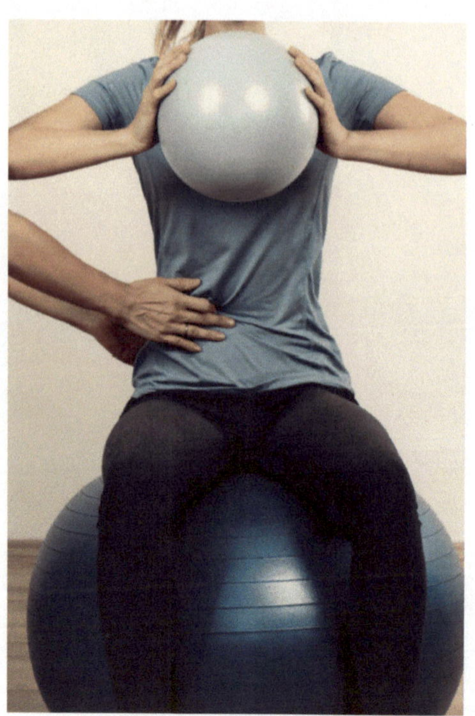

One significant benefitof Pilates exercises is its ability to strengthen the back muscles and promote spinal health,reducing the risk of low back pain and improving overall posture. This targeted approach to strengthening the back plays a vital role in injury prevention and supports a healthy, pain-free spine.

Overall, Pilates exercises provide a comprehensive approachto body conditioning, addressing muscle strength, flexibility, and balance to promote optimal physical well-being. With modifications available for different fitness levels and individual needs, Pilates can be tailored to accommodate a wide range of practitioners, ensuring that everyone may benefit from its principles.

By implementing a structured Pilates routine that gradually builds strength and stability over time, individuals could progress effectively and safely in their practice. Incorporating breathing techniques into Pilates exercises further enhances the mind-body connection, fostering mindfulness and enhancing the overall experience of movement.

Nearly every Pilates exercise involves pointing or flexing your feet. Footwork on the reformer offers a unique and effective approach to improving foot and lower extremity biomechanics, as well as enhancing foot flexibility and strength. With consistent practice, Pilates can help alleviate and even eliminate foot pain.

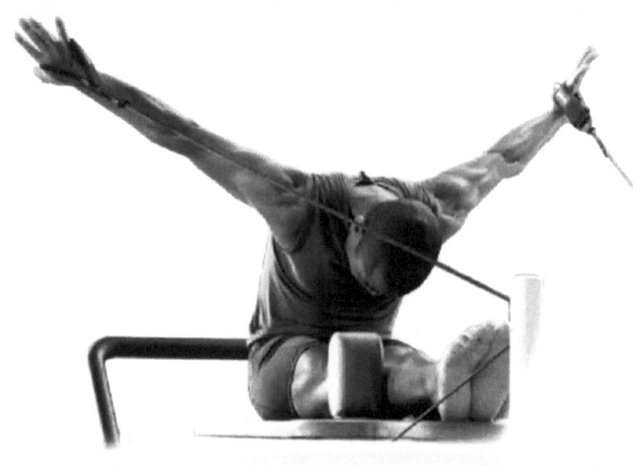

In conclusion, the adaptability of Pilates exercises makes it suitable for individuals with hypermobility. The controlled and intentional movements could help improve joint stability and support joint health. This adaptability confirms the inclusive nature of Pilates, making it a versatile and effective form of exercise for individuals with diverse needs and abilities.

CHAPTER 14

SUSTAINABLE MOVEMENT: EMBRACING PILATES PRINCIPLES

This chapter aims to inspire you as individuals to take proactive steps towards sustained health, fitness, and overall vitality for a fulfilling and healthy lifestyle.

Embracing the core principles of alignment, stability, and strength in Pilates routines is key to developing a strong and resilient body. By incorporating these foundational elements into each workout session, individuals can reap the benefits of improved posture, enhanced muscular endurance, and increased overall physical function.

PILATES PRINCIPLES

1. CONCENTRATION
2. BREATHING
3. CENTRING
4. CONTROL
5. PRECISION
6. FLUID AND FLOWING MOVEMENTS
7. ISOLATION
8. ROUTINE

To foster a long-term commitment to improving physical well-being, Pilates serves as a valuable tool for individuals seeking sustainable health and fitness practices. The transformative impact of Pilates on overall health and vitality is evident in the strength, flexibility, and body awareness that practitioners cultivate through consistent practice.

Pilates exercises are highly adaptable to individual needs and goals, making it accessible to individuals of all fitness levels and physical abilities. By integrating Pilates principles into everyday movements, individuals can enhance their functionality and movement efficiency in various aspects of their daily lives.

We hope you gained some insight into the positive effects of a dedicated Pilates practice on overall well-being. If you would like more guidance on establishing a sustainable movement routine with Pilates, you can contact us to help you create a structured and effective plan for incorporating Pilates into your lifestyle for long-term health benefits.

Pilates stands as a time-tested movement practice that prioritises quality and control in every exercise. By exploring the foundations of Pilates, individuals can appreciate its focus on precise movements, proper alignment, and core engagement, culminating in improved movement efficiency and body awareness.

The benefits of Pilates exercises in promoting stability and strength cannot be overstated. Whether targeting core muscles, enhancing muscle tone, or improving overall body strength, Pilates offers a well-rounded approach to physical fitness that fosters stability, balance, and functional strength.

Described as a sustainable and holistic approach to fitness, Pilates encompasses not only the physical aspect of exercise but also mental well-being and mindfulness. Its adaptability for individuals of varying fitness levels makes it an inclusive practice that can be tailored to meet the needs and goals of each practitioner.

FURTHER READING

Reference & useful pages

Mikkonen, J., et. al. "A Survey of Musculoskeletal Injury among Ashtanga Vinyasa Yoga Practitioners." Int J Yoga Therap, 2008; 18(1):59–64. doi:10.17761/ijyt.18.1.I0748p25k2558v77

Kumar, R. A. & Chakkaravarthy, S. "A Survey on Yogic Posture Recognition." IEEE, 2023;11:11183–11223. doi: 10.1109/ACCESS.2023.3240769

"Yoga More Dangerous than Previously Thought, Scientists Say." The Telegraph, 2017. www.telegraph.co.uk/ news/2017/06/28/yogamore-dangerous-previously-thought- scientists-say/. Accessed 30 Aug 2024.

Nicholis, K. "Why I Started Pilates (and Stopped Yoga)." Happiful Magazine, 2023. happiful.com/why-i-started-pilates- and-stopped-yoga. Accessed 30 Aug 2024.

Gajadharsingh, G. The Health Equation. https://www.thehealthequation.co.uk/ Accessed 30 Aug 2024

"What can Pilates 'Lateral Breathing' do for me?." Pilates Blogger UK, 2020. https://pilatesblogger.co.uk/what-can- pilates-lateral-breathing-do-for-me/ Accessed 30 Aug 2024

Beditation - Pilates breathwork exercises for everyday and/or chronic pain on The Hope Centre UK APP - iTunes, Spotify- https://beditation.co.uk/

Useful references:

Hypermobility Syndromes Association.
www.hypermobility.org

HMSA Book - Understanding hEDS and HSD by Claire Smith

HMSA publications - trifold leaflets, 'What's the Connection' Posters, Educators guide etc.

HMSA website - Explaining An HMS To Friends and Family

Stickman communications website - https://stickmancommunications.co.uk/products/

Sunflower lanyards for hidden disabilities - https://hiddendisabilitiesstore.com/shop/sunflower-lanyards.html
Links between hypermobility & anxiety:
Eccles, J. What is the link between joint hypermobility and anxiety? YouTube, 2018.
https://www.youtube.com/watch?v=Mjo7rdAv5ps&t=31s

Eccles, J. Anxiety and Hypermobility. Ac Med Sci, 2020. https:// www.youtube.com/watch?v=XYJsXaqixBY

Eccles, J. et al. "Brain structure and joint hypermobility: relevance to the expression of psychiatric symptoms." Br J Psychiatry 2012;200(6): 508-509. doi:10.1192/bjp.bp.111.092460

Csecs, J. L., et al. "Variant Connective Tissue (Joint Hypermobility) and Dysautonomia Are Associated with Multimorbidity at the Intersection between Physical and Psychological Health." American Journal of Medical Genetics Part C: Seminars in Medical Genetics, 2021;187(4):500-509. doi:10.1002/ajmg.c.31957.